HORMONE RESET

DIET

FOR NOVICES

Enriched Recipes, Foods, Meal Plan &
Procedures For Hormonal Balance,
Weight Management, Metabolism
Healing And More

DR. MATEO GABRIEL

DISCLAIMER

The information in this book is only meant to be used for general reading. In any way, the author and publisher do not promise or represent that the information in this work is full, correct, reliable, appropriate, or available. This includes any warranties that are expressed or implied. Because of this, you should only rely on this material at your own risk.

This book is not meant to replace professional help. If you have any questions about a subject, you should always get help from a qualified expert. The author and distributor of this book are not responsible for how the information in it is used or abused.

TABLE OF CONTENTS

CHAPTER ONE

INTRODUCTION TO HORMONE RESET DIET

KNOWLEDGE OF HORMONES

A thorough grasp of the complex role hormones play in the human body forms the basis of the Hormone Reset Diet. Hormones are essentially chemical messengers that control a wide range of physiological activities, including mood, reproduction, energy balance, metabolism, and energy balance. These signaling molecules are produced by several organs, including the pancreas, thyroid, and adrenal glands.

They enter the circulation and reach target cells, where they alter their activity.

PHYSIOLOGICAL ROLES OF HORMONES

Every hormone has a distinct purpose, and homeostasis depends on the proper coordination of their functions. For example, the thyroid gland produces thyroid hormones, which are essential for controlling metabolism, and the pancreas produces insulin, which is vital for maintaining blood sugar levels. Examples of sex hormones that influence reproductive processes and contribute to the development of secondary sexual features are testosterone and estrogens.

The importance of preserving a precise equilibrium is shown by the complex dance of hormones. A hormonal imbalance in these messengers can cause a series of health problems, as acknowledged by the Hormone Reset Diet. Hormone functions are interrelated, so changes in one can have a significant impact on overall health. For optimum health and vigor, hormone balance must be achieved and maintained.

THE SIGNIFICANCE OF HORMONAL BALANCE

When one considers how hormone balance affects weight and general health, the significance of this becomes quite clear. Hormones are essential for controlling hunger, metabolism, and fat accumulation. For example, abnormalities in insulin secretion may result in a rise in fat accumulation, hence exacerbating weight gain and insulin resistance. Chronic stress can cause overeating and weight gain because cortisol, the stress hormone generated by the adrenal glands, affects appetite and fat storage.

HOW HORMONES IMPACT HEALTH AND WEIGHT

Hormonal changes can also impact mood and energy levels, which can impact lifestyle decisions like eating and exercise routines. Hormonal imbalances can lead to desires for high-fat or sugary meals, which can make it difficult to stick to a nutritious diet. Understanding the complex relationship between hormones and weight, the Hormone Reset Diet seeks to reset and optimize these chemical messengers for long-term, sustainable health benefits.

The Hormone Reset Diet is based on a thorough comprehension of the intricate realm of hormones and their roles. Understanding how crucial it is to preserve a fine balance, the diet aims to address how hormone imbalances affect weight and general health.

CHAPTER TWO

SYNOPSIS OF THE HORMONE RESET DIET

THE HORMONE RESET DIET: WHAT IS IT?

The ultimate purpose of the Hormone Reset Diet is to promote general health and well-being by optimizing and rebalancing the body's hormonal levels through nutrition. It is based on the idea that variations in energy, weight gain, and other health problems might be caused by hormone imbalances, which are frequently caused by different lifestyle circumstances. The diet places a strong emphasis on the necessity of careful timing and choosing nutrients to reset and regulate hormones, which will boost energy levels, metabolism, and weight management.

HISTORY AND ORIGIN

The emerging understanding of the profound influence hormones have on the body's operation is responsible for the origins and evolution of the Hormone Reset Diet. The idea gained popularity because of the 2015 publication of "The Hormone Reset Diet," a book by Harvard-trained physician and author Dr. Sara Gottfried that explores the relationship between hormones and how they affect mood, weight, and general health. Drawing from both scientific knowledge and her clinical experience, Dr. Gottfried's approach aims to restore hormonal balance through focused dietary interventions and lifestyle modifications.

IMPORTANT IDEAS

The Hormone Reset Diet's main tenets center on choosing the right nutrients, timing meals, and making lifestyle adjustments. One of the main principles involves following three separate stages, each lasting roughly three to four days, and implementing particular food regimes that target various hormonal systems. For example, the initial stage concentrates on restoring insulin levels, frequently through lowering carbohydrate consumption and placing an emphasis on complete, nutrient-dense diets. Phases that follow focus on sex hormones and cortisol, adjusting the diet to meet the specific requirements of each hormonal system.

When it comes to choosing nutrients, the diet places a strong emphasis on including a range of vibrant veggies, healthy fats, and premium proteins. These nutrient-dense foods have been selected because they may help maintain general health and hormonal balance. The diet also promotes the consumption of particular foods, such as those high in fiber, antioxidants, and omega-3 fatty acids, which are known to have a favorable effect on hormones.

In addition to dietary modifications, the Hormone Reset Diet promotes lifestyle changes to enhance the nutritional benefits. Regular physical activity, stress reduction, and adequate sleep are essential since they all have a significant impact on hormone control. Particular emphasis is placed on sleep's effects on growth hormone and cortisol levels, underscoring the relationship between lifestyle choices and hormonal health.

The Hormone Reset Diet addresses hormonal imbalances through deliberate food adjustments and lifestyle changes, providing a comprehensive approach to health. This nutritional approach, which is based on the knowledge of the complex interaction between hormones and general health, attempts to provide people the ability to manage their health by promoting hormonal balance. The Hormone Reset Diet, which is based on the ideas of a balanced diet, intentional meal planning, and holistic lifestyle practices, provides a thorough roadmap for anyone looking to maximize their hormonal health and attain long-term well-being.

CHAPTER THREE

HORMONE RESET DIET BENEFITS

MAINTAINING WEIGHT

The Hormone Reset Diet has become more well-known due to its possible advantages in controlling weight. This method acknowledges the complex interplay between hormones and weight. Advocates of the Hormone Reset Diet assert that it can assist control of hormones like insulin, cortisol, and leptin, which are important for metabolism and fat storage, by concentrating on particular dietary adjustments and lifestyle changes. Through focused nutritional therapies that address hormonal imbalances, people may achieve longer-lasting weight loss and improved weight maintenance. A healthy weight is supported by the emphasis on full, nutrient-dense foods and the decrease in processed and refined carbs.

ENHANCED LEVELS OF ENERGY

An important benefit of doing a Hormone Reset Diet is that it may increase energy levels. The diet promotes the consumption of foods that help blood sugar levels stay steady, avoiding the crashes and spikes that come with eating a lot of refined carbohydrates and processed sugars. People who prioritize lean proteins, healthy fats, and complex carbs may feel energized for the day. Avoiding meals that deplete energy will help maintain a more steady and balanced energy supply, which can lessen fatigue and increase general vitality.

ENDOCRINE HEALTH

Supporting hormonal health is a major focus of the Hormone Reset Diet. The body uses hormones as messengers to regulate several physiological processes, such as mood, metabolism, and reproductive activities. The goal of this diet is to normalize hormones by treating issues like cortisol levels and insulin resistance. For instance, the diet aims to increase insulin sensitivity by limiting the consumption of processed foods and refined sugars, which may lower the risk of insulin-related health problems. The Hormone Reset Diet also promotes general hormonal balance by including foods high in vital nutrients, which enhances long-term health and well-being.

MENTAL FOCUS AND CLARITY

An increase in focus and mental clarity has been mentioned as another advantage of the hormone reset diet. There is rising interest in the relationship between nutrition and cognition, and proponents of the Hormone Reset nutrition contend that specific dietary patterns can improve brain function. The diet delivers vital vitamins and minerals that are necessary for optimum brain function by emphasizing nutrient-dense foods. Additionally, blood sugar stabilization—achieved by avoiding high-glycemic foods—may support prolonged concentration and mental focus. Proponents of the Hormone Reset Diet contend that it may improve cognitive function, while individual results may differ.

The Hormone Reset Diet provides a comprehensive strategy for overall health and wellness, addressing issues like mental clarity, energy levels, weight control, and hormonal balance. People may see gains in these areas by concentrating on full, nutrient-dense foods and implementing lifestyle changes, which could result in a more sustainable and balanced approach to overall health. Individual results may differ, as with any diet plan, so it's important to speak with medical professionals before making big dietary adjustments, particularly for people with pre-existing medical concerns.

CHAPTER FOUR
PRIMARY HORMONES
INSULIN

The pancreatic beta cells secrete the vital hormone insulin, which is responsible for controlling blood glucose levels. The body converts carbs into glucose when we eat them, which raises blood sugar levels. Insulin helps cells absorb glucose so they may either use it as fuel or store it as glycogen in the muscles and liver. Blood glucose levels rise in diseases like diabetes because the body either produces insufficient insulin (Type 1) or the cells develop resistance to its effects (Type 2).

Ensuring optimal insulin action is essential for maintaining overall metabolic health.

INTISOLA

The adrenal glands create cortisol, also known as the "stress hormone." Stress, both mental and physical, causes it to release. By activating energy reserves, inhibiting non-essential processes like the immune system, and accelerating the metabolism of carbohydrates, proteins, and lipids, cortisol aids the body in adjusting to stress. On the other hand, persistently high cortisol levels can have detrimental impacts on health, such as weakened immune systems, weight gain, and irregular sleep patterns. Cortisol levels must be kept within a healthy range by managing stress and implementing constructive coping techniques.

SLEEPING

The hormone leptin, which is generated by fat cells, is essential for controlling hunger and energy balance. When the body has enough fat reserves, it signals the brain through its action on the hypothalamus. Elevated leptin levels aid in weight maintenance by decreasing appetite and boosting energy expenditure. However, leptin resistance, which occurs when the body no longer reacts to leptin signals effectively, can occur in people with illnesses like obesity, which can result in overeating and weight increase.

THYMOSIN

The stomach produces ghrelin, also known as the "hunger hormone," which increases appetite. Usually, ghrelin levels increase before meals and fall following consumption. It encourages food intake and energy storage in contrast to leptin. Ghrelin levels are influenced by several factors, including stress, lack of sleep, and irregular eating patterns. These factors may exacerbate weight-related problems. To control appetite and keep a healthy weight, one must comprehend how ghrelin interacts with other hormones.

THYROID SUBSTANCES

Thyroxine (T4) and triiodothyronine (T3) are two examples of thyroid hormones that are produced by the thyroid gland and are essential for controlling metabolism. They affect the body's temperature, energy consumption, and heart rate, among other physiological functions. Energy levels, metabolism, and general well-being can all be significantly impacted by conditions like hyperthyroidism (excessive thyroid hormone production) and hypothyroidism (insufficient thyroid hormone production). Maintaining a healthy metabolism and avoiding associated health problems require balancing thyroid hormone levels.

The key hormones—thyroid hormones, cortisol, leptin, ghrelin, and insulin—cooperate to control many facets of metabolism, energy balance, and general health. Promoting well-being and preventing hormonal imbalances, which can lead to a variety of health problems, need an understanding of these substances' roles and the variables that affect their levels.

CHAPTER FIVE

HORMONAL DISPROPORTIONS

TYPICAL CAUSES

A multitude of frequent causes can give rise to hormonal imbalances, which are defined as disturbances of the delicate hormonal balance in the body. Stress is a common component because it causes the body to generate cortisol, which can disrupt the levels of other hormones. Furthermore, eating is very important since hormone synthesis and regulation are impacted by inadequate nutrition and an imbalance of vital nutrients. Hormonal imbalances can also be caused by environmental pollutants, such as the endocrine-disrupting substances included in some plastics and pesticides.

Hormonal variations are also greatly influenced by age and stage of life. Hormonal changes are normal during key life stages including puberty, pregnancy, and menopause, but they can also be linked to imbalances that cause a variety of symptoms. Hormonal imbalances can also be caused by medical illnesses such as thyroid problems and polycystic ovarian syndrome (PCOS). The endocrine system's regular operation may be interfered with by certain disorders, which may affect the secretion and control of hormones.

SYMPTOMS AND INDICES

Understanding the telltale signs and symptoms of hormone imbalances is essential for prompt management and intervention. Although each person's symptoms may present differently, frequent markers include exhaustion, mood swings, changes in appetite, weight gain or loss, and irregular sleep habits. Hormonal imbalances can also be connected to changes in libido and irregular menstruation in women, as well as skin conditions like acne and dryness. In addition, people may have trouble concentrating, lose their hair, and become more sensitive to heat or cold. These symptoms might all be signs of hormonal imbalances that are interfering with different body processes.

EFFECT ON WELL-BEING

Hormonal imbalances have a significant effect on health that affects many different bodily systems. Hormones are essential for controlling immunological responses, mood, metabolism, and reproductive processes. Therefore, imbalances in hormones can cause mental health problems, metabolic abnormalities, and problems with reproduction. For example, abnormalities in sex hormones such as testosterone and estrogen can impact menstrual cycles, fertility, and sperm production in women, and can also lead to reproductive issues.

Hormonal abnormalities can also impact the chance of developing chronic illnesses like osteoporosis, diabetes, and cardiovascular diseases. Because the endocrine system, which produces and regulates hormones, is linked to other physiological systems, changes in hormone levels may have a domino impact on one's general health. Hormonal abnormalities can have an impact on mental health as well; disorders like anxiety and depression are exacerbated by these imbalances.

Treating hormonal imbalances requires an awareness of the typical causes, symptoms, and indicators as well as the wider effects on health. For effective prevention, diagnosis, and management of hormone imbalances, a comprehensive approach that takes into account lifestyle variables, environmental effects, and individual health history is necessary. By having a thorough understanding of these ideas, both individuals and healthcare professionals can work to promote general well-being and restore hormonal homeostasis.

CHAPTER SIX

HORMONE RESET DIET: HOW TO USE IT

CHANGING YOUR NUTRITION

The core tenet of the hormone reset diet is that you may restore your body's hormonal equilibrium by making deliberate dietary adjustments. The idea is that some lifestyle choices, including stress and unhealthy eating patterns, can throw off the balance of hormones, which can result in weight gain and other health problems. People who follow the Hormone Reset Diet want to achieve overall health and harmony in their lives.

COMPARING PROCESSED AND WHOLE FOODS

The emphasis on real foods over processed substitutes is a cornerstone of the Hormone Reset Diet. Whole foods include vital nutrients devoid of artificial additives, preservatives, and added sugars that are frequently present in processed foods. Examples of these foods include fruits, vegetables, lean proteins, and whole grains. The idea is to minimize the intake of processed, inflammatory foods that might upset the endocrine system, and instead fuel the body with natural, nutrient-dense foods that support hormonal balance and metabolic function.

THE SIGNIFICANCE OF TIMING NUTRIENTS

A crucial component of the Hormone Reset Diet is nutrient timing, which addresses the timing of your nutrient intake throughout the day. The idea acknowledges the critical role hormone fluctuations play in energy control and metabolism. People can maximize their hormone levels and encourage muscular growth and fat-burning by timing their dietary intake. Consuming carbohydrates, for instance, can improve nutritional absorption and boost glycogen replenishment during times of elevated insulin sensitivity, such as during exercise.

PLANNING AND PREPARING MEALS

Planning and preparing meals in advance is essential to following the Hormone Reset Diet properly. Meal preparation in advance enables people to choose carefully what they eat and how much of it. It also aids in avoiding rash, unhealthful food decisions. Meal preparation at home allows you more control over ingredients and cooking techniques, which makes it easier to follow the guidelines of the diet.

CHAPTER SEVEN

ESSENTIAL MINERALS FOR HORMONE BALANCE

VITAL MINERALS AND VITAMINS

Essential minerals and vitamins are vital for preserving the body's hormonal equilibrium. These micronutrients participate in a variety of enzymatic processes related to hormone synthesis, metabolism, and control as cofactors and catalysts. For example, it is well known that vitamin D is necessary for the synthesis of steroid hormones, such as testosterone and estrogen.

Similar to this, deficits in minerals like zinc and selenium can throw off the hormonal balance because these elements are essential for thyroid function. The proper balance of B vitamins, especially B6 and B12, is also linked to the control of hormones like progesterone and estrogen.

THE FATTY ACIDS OMEGA-3

For hormonal balance, omega-3 fatty acids—which are mostly present in walnuts, flaxseeds, and fatty fish—are crucial. These fatty acids support the fluidity and integrity of cell membranes and are the building blocks of hormones. They are essential for the synthesis of prostaglandins, which are hormone-like molecules that control blood coagulation and inflammation. Reduced inflammation and enhanced insulin sensitivity are two benefits of omega-3 fatty acids, particularly docosahexaenoic acid (DHA) and eicosapentaenoic acid (EPA), both of which are essential for maintaining hormonal balance.

OXIDIZERS

Antioxidants, which include various vitamins like C and E and minerals like selenium, shield the body from the damaging effects of free radicals. Because oxidative stress damages cells, including those involved in hormone production and regulation, it can upset the balance of hormones. Free radicals are countered by antioxidants, reducing the possibility of cellular damage and promoting hormonal balance in general. Vitamin E, for instance, has been linked to preventing oxidative damage to the ovaries, which may be especially important for female reproductive hormones.

TISSUE

Fruits, vegetables, whole grains, and legumes are good sources of fiber, which has a variety of functions in regulating hormones. Sufficient consumption of fiber promotes gut health, and better hormone regulation is associated with a thriving gut flora.

By reducing the rate at which glucose is absorbed, fiber also helps to regulate blood sugar by averting insulin surges. This is especially important for diseases like insulin resistance, where hormone balance depends on steady blood sugar levels. Furthermore, fiber aids in the elimination of excess hormones, avoiding their build-up and possible endocrine system disruption.

The interaction of fiber, antioxidants, omega-3 fatty acids, and important vitamins and minerals is critical to preserving hormonal equilibrium. These nutrients support general health, shield the body from oxidative stress, and aid in the production, regulation, and metabolism of hormones. To foster hormonal equilibrium and prevent imbalances that may result in several health problems, a diet rich in nutrients and well-balanced is crucial.

CHAPTER EIGHT

METHODS FOR MAINTAINING HORMONE BALANCE

STRESS MANAGEMENT

The body's hormones are largely regulated by how well stress is managed. Cortisol, a hormone that can upset the delicate hormonal balance when raised for prolonged periods, is released as a result of chronic stress. Deep breathing exercises, yoga, and mindfulness meditation are among the techniques that have been demonstrated to lower stress and, as a result, support cortisol regulation. Through the implementation of these strategies in their daily lives, individuals can lessen the detrimental effects of stress on their hormone health.

GOOD SLEEP

Hormonal balance depends on getting enough good sleep. The body goes through vital processes of regeneration and repair when we sleep, and any disturbances in this cycle can impact the synthesis of hormones. Growth hormone, for example, is mostly released during prolonged sleep and aids in muscle growth and tissue repair. Conversely, lack of sleep has been connected to elevated cortisol levels and abnormalities in insulin sensitivity. Supporting hormonal balance requires establishing a regular sleep schedule and setting up a comfortable sleeping environment.

EXERCISE AND HORMONAL HEALTH

A key component of hormonal health is regular physical activity. Exercise has a significant effect on several hormones, such as sex hormones, insulin, and cortisol. Specifically, resistance exercise has been linked to higher levels of growth hormone and testosterone synthesis, two essential hormones for preserving muscle mass and general health. Conversely, overdoing endurance exercise can raise cortisol levels, which highlights the significance of an individualized and balanced approach to exercise. Optimizing hormonal health requires finding the ideal mix between aerobic and resistance training.

HYDRATION

An essential but frequently disregarded component of hormonal homeostasis is hydration. The endocrine system depends on water to function properly, which helps hormones move throughout the body. Hormone synthesis and secretion can be affected by dehydration, which can result in imbalances. Drinking enough water helps the kidneys eliminate extra hormones and toxins, which keeps them from building up. Furthermore, maintaining proper hydration during exercise is essential for regulating body temperature and avoiding imbalances caused by stress. Sustaining a steady and adequate quantity of water is an easy but effective way to support hormonal health in general.

Attaining hormonal balance necessitates a comprehensive strategy that includes stress reduction, restful sleep, consistent exercise, and adequate water. Through the use of these lifestyle choices, people can establish a conducive atmosphere for the endocrine system, thereby cultivating hormonal balance and augmenting general health.

CHAPTER NINE
EXAMPLES OF MENUS
BREAKFAST CONCEPTS

A hearty and well-balanced breakfast provides the necessary fuel and nutrients for the body to function at its best throughout the day. A balanced start is guaranteed when a range of dietary categories are included. Complex carbohydrates found in whole grains like oats and whole wheat toast help to maintain energy levels throughout the morning. In addition to improving satiety, pairing these with high-protein foods like

Greek yogurt or eggs helps maintain and repair muscle.

Fruits also provide essential vitamins and antioxidants. A fruit salad or smoothie that contains berries, bananas, and spinach will give it a tasty and nutrient-dense boost. A vegetable omelet with a side of avocados provides a combination of fiber, healthy fats, and important micronutrients for those who prefer a heartier meal.

LUNCH AND DINNER OPTIONS

Lunch and dinner present opportunities to create well-rounded meals that satisfy both taste and nutritional needs. A diverse array of vegetables should form a significant portion of these meals, offering fiber, vitamins, and minerals. Lean protein sources, such as grilled chicken, fish, or legumes, contribute to muscle health and aid in achieving a feeling of fullness.

Whole grains like quinoa or brown rice provide complex carbohydrates, releasing energy gradually and sustaining you throughout the day. Incorporating healthy fats from sources like olive oil, nuts, or avocado not only adds flavor but also supports various bodily functions. Stir-fries with colorful vegetables, lean protein, and a light sauce, or grain bowls with a mix of veggies, protein, and a wholesome grain, are excellent options for both lunch and dinner.

SNACK SUGGESTIONS

Snacking can be an opportunity to nourish your body between meals and prevent energy slumps. Opting for nutrient-dense snacks helps maintain steady blood sugar levels and prevents overeating during main meals. A handful of nuts, such as almonds or walnuts, provides a satisfying combination of healthy fats, protein, and fiber.

Greek yogurt with a drizzle of honey and a sprinkle of berries offers a sweet yet nutritious option. Vegetable sticks with hummus or guacamole make for a crunchy and satisfying snack that's rich in vitamins and minerals.

CHAPTER TEN

RECIPES FOR HORMONE BALANCE

HORMONE-FRIENDLY SMOOTHIES

Creating hormone-friendly smoothies involves incorporating ingredients that support hormonal balance and overall well-being. These smoothies are designed to provide essential nutrients that contribute to hormonal health. Start with a base of leafy greens such as kale or spinach, which are rich in vitamins and minerals. Add fruits like berries, which contain antioxidants and fiber that help regulate blood sugar levels.

To further enhance hormone balance, include healthy fats like avocados or coconut oil. These fats are crucial for the production of hormones and can help stabilize energy levels throughout the day. Consider adding a scoop of protein powder, preferably a plant-based option, to support muscle health and maintain a steady release of energy.

BALANCED MEALS

Balanced meals play a pivotal role in maintaining hormone equilibrium. Aim for a combination of macronutrients in each meal protein, carbohydrates, and fats. Include lean proteins like chicken, fish, or tofu, which provide amino acids necessary for hormone synthesis. Carbohydrates from whole grains, vegetables, and fruits contribute to stable blood sugar levels, preventing hormonal fluctuations.

Incorporate healthy fats, such as those found in olive oil, nuts, and seeds, to support the production of hormones and aid in nutrient absorption. Additionally, prioritize a variety of colorful vegetables on your plate to ensure a broad spectrum of vitamins and minerals. This diverse nutrient intake can positively impact hormone function and overall health.

HORMONE RESET SNACKS

Hormone reset snacks are convenient, satisfying options that help regulate energy levels and prevent hormonal imbalances between meals. Opt for snacks that combine protein and healthy fats to promote satiety and stabilize blood sugar. Greek yogurt with a handful of almonds or an apple with nut butter is excellent choices.

Consider incorporating snacks rich in fiber, such as raw vegetables with hummus or a small serving of berries, to support digestive health and regulate insulin levels. Avoid processed snacks high in refined sugars, as they can contribute to hormonal spikes and crashes. Instead, choose whole, nutrient-dense options that nourish your body and contribute to hormonal balance throughout the day.

CHAPTER ELEVEN

OVERCOMING CHALLENGES

DEALING WITH CRAVINGS

Dealing with cravings is a universal challenge that many individuals encounter on their journey towards healthier living. Cravings often emerge as intense desires for specific foods, high in sugar, salt, or unhealthy fats. To effectively tackle cravings, it is crucial to understand their origins and triggers. Cravings can be influenced by various factors, including emotional states, stress, hormonal fluctuations, and even environmental cues. Recognizing the root cause of cravings allows individuals to develop targeted strategies for overcoming them.

UNDERSTANDING CRAVINGS

Understanding cravings involves delving into the psychological and physiological aspects of these urges. On a psychological level, cravings may be linked to emotional needs, such as stress relief or comfort-seeking. Physiologically, the body's response to certain foods can create addictive patterns, making it challenging to break free from unhealthy eating habits. By acknowledging the multifaceted nature of cravings, individuals can adopt a holistic approach to address both the emotional and physical components, fostering a more sustainable path to overcoming these challenges.

STRATEGIES FOR OVERCOMING CRAVINGS

Strategies for overcoming cravings encompass a range of techniques aimed at managing both the psychological and physiological aspects of this obstacle. Cognitive-behavioral strategies, such as identifying and challenging negative thought patterns related to cravings, can empower individuals to regain control over their eating habits. Additionally, incorporating mindful eating practices, such as savoring each bite and paying attention to hunger and fullness cues, can promote a healthier relationship with food. Substituting healthier alternatives for craving-inducing foods and engaging in regular physical activity also play integral roles in curbing cravings and promoting overall well-being.

SOCIAL AND LIFESTYLE CHALLENGES

Social and lifestyle challenges further compound the difficulties of adopting a healthier lifestyle. Navigating social events, where unhealthy food options are often abundant, requires a combination of planning and assertiveness. Communicating dietary preferences and goals with friends and family can foster understanding and support. Bringing nutritious snacks to gatherings and actively seeking out healthier menu options are effective strategies for maintaining dietary discipline amidst social temptations.

TRAVELING ON THE HORMONE RESET DIET

Traveling on the Hormone Reset Diet adds an extra layer of complexity to the challenge of adhering to a specific eating plan. Planning by researching and identifying hormone-friendly dining options at travel destinations is crucial. Packing portable, nutrient-dense snacks can serve as a convenient alternative to unhealthy airport or roadside fare. Maintaining consistency in meal timing and incorporating physical activity while traveling can contribute to hormone balance and overall well-being.

Overcoming challenges related to cravings, social situations, and lifestyle adjustments requires a comprehensive and adaptable approach. By understanding the roots of cravings, adopting effective strategies, and proactively addressing social and lifestyle influences, individuals can navigate these hurdles successfully on their journey to improved health and well-being.